ACKNOWLEDGMENTS

Many thanks to Jessica Stanton, an experienced writer, for assistance in writing the book, especially with character and story development and working to ensure that the publication met its three main objectives. My karate instructor and best friend, Stuart Rowe, provided valuable feedback throughout the process, and from day one continued to remind me that the endeavor is for a noble cause. Jovita Robertson, my niece, was enthusiastic about the undertaking from the start and helped in various ways, not the least of which was to keep me excited too. And special thanks to friends and relatives who gave me encouragement to write the book.

This book is dedicated to my grandson, Kordye Turner III, who I affectionately call K3, for inspiring me to wake up each day and try to make the most of it, even on my worst days.

PROLOGUE

Raise your hand if you like pain! If you raised your hand, please put it down, you look silly! Let's be honest, pain sucks! However, the never-ending, internal power struggle between our able mind and unwilling body, is a classic story for most peoples' lives. Insidiously, the balance of power between ability and pain gradually changes over time. This book is part of the story of two brothers, Pain and Able. It is about their journey together through the ups and downs of life while controlling the same body. What could possibly go wrong?

In youth, Able is our hero, and we sure love to put him on a pedestal, don't we? But as aging occurs, all too soon, Pain becomes a dominant controller of our lives. And then Pain swiftly kicks that pedestal, right out from under ability, leaving us (sometimes literally) sprawled on the floor. Able, who in youth usually ignored Pain, is now roughly pushed aside by Pain.

Since Pain hasn't been able to command respect in the past, he will demand it now. No more Mr. nice guy. No more being treated like a nobody. Pain is now intent on going from zero to hero! It's time for Able to grow up and accept that they are different now before it's too late for both of them! Optimism be damned; it is time to be practical. It is time for a reality check! It is time for Able to accept what is, instead of what he wants it to be.

But change is hard for all of us, isn't it? Because that thought can be so overwhelming, I have written this short story, with three main objectives:

1. Remind you, dear reader, that you are not alone in your struggle to live with pain! The timeless and universal truth is that aging brings all types of body pain. It's inevitable. We must listen to our bodies and adjust or suffer the consequences.

2. Provide a lighter, more amusing perspective, and perhaps acceptance of our condition through the Pain and Able saga. However, we all know that pain, especially severe pain, is not very funny; rather it's a bitch!

3. And finally, to a lesser degree, to point out that the side effects of statins, *cholesterol-lowering drugs*, can be devastating to some people, especially athletes.

So, shall we start a journey together?

CHAPTER 1

One lovely spring day, in the prime of their lives, a pensive Pain looked over at his brother Able and said, "We need to take care of ourselves; otherwise we are not going to last too long." Pain had noticed lately, that they were getting a little older, and the recent doctor's visit had greatly concerned him. Pain was smart enough to recognize they were mortal and wanted to extend said mortality as long as possible.

Able looked at his brother drolly and blew his brother off with a wave of the hand. "Yes, yes, you're right. I have been thinking about that lately, and I think I have come up with a solution. Did I tell you I'm going to start working out to become very fit and eventually earn a black belt in karate? It's something I have always wanted to do!

A look of horror crossed Pains already tight face. He replied incredulously, "You want to do what?! We just had what the cardiologist called "a small heart attack!" You might consider that inconsequential, but I don't. It is like saying we had a small nuclear bomb dropped on us! We also had a stent put in one of the main arteries leading to our heart. We are supposed to be walking on eggshells now, not crashing around like a bull in a china shop!"

Pain let out a frustrated huff, unable to comprehend his brother's carelessness.

Able rolled his eyes, thinking his overly cautious brother was overacting again. "Yes, but we had a total cholesterol level of over 300! Also, we weren't taking good care of ourselves, eating anything we wanted, and not staying in shape. Too much of that tasty, albeit greasy, food I guess."

Able sidled up to Pain and said in a cajoling tone. "But we can change that! Remember they started us on a statin drug to lower our cholesterol? We have a chance now to change everything about our health for the better! And improve and live longer." Able wrapped his arm around Pain's shoulder and gave him a quick squeeze. "Trust me, Pal, we need this."

Pain looked dubiously at his brother. "I'm not ready for any type of rigorous training program, Able, and I don't think you are either. You must realize that we are 43 years old now! Don't you think is a little late for that? If we were going to do that, we should have started long ago."

Able looked at Pain as if he was a pitiful, ignorant child, and shook his head. "It's never too late to improve one's health, Pain. Trust me. Why are you always trying to rain on my parade anyway? Coward?"

Pain raised an eyebrow at Able "Because I want to live a long and comfortable life, underscore comfortable. Why don't you?"

Able ignored Pain's question and tersely responded "Oh,

shut-up Pain. Enough already! You're always so negative. Why can't you just go along with this?"

Pain chuckled wryly and retorted, "And you're always so positive! You believe we can do anything with that can-do attitude. Your optimism and confidence are going to get us hurt someday, and bad! I don't want that! When we were much younger, we could get away with a lot of strenuous physical activity. We certainly played enough sports. If you remember, I rarely complained then. But we are much older now, and I'm not sure you've gotten much wiser." Able stared, unbelieving at Pain's sharp observation, while Pain continued, oblivious.

"All the things we used to be able to do, I don't think we should do anymore. And it's my job to remind you that too much physical activity will do us more harm than good. There are a lot of problems that we could develop that will cause me to complain, attempting to save us. I will do anything to help us have a long and happy life. One that is not full of pain and medical problems!"

Able sighed deeply and pleadingly replied with "I got your point Pain. I just think if we work to stay fit and take care of our body, that our body will take care of us. I want to live a long and happy life too. Who wouldn't? But to me, it's never too late to do the right thing. It is also my job to help us live the best possible life, as long as we can! I just believe my optimistic approach is much better than your pessimistic one. Perhaps it was my reluctance not to have pain and discomfort from working out, that caused our heart problem in the first place. But it's time to change." Able crossed his arms over his chest a little self smugly and said smilingly, "I don't believe my willing and able mind has ever let you down, Mr. Body Pain. Anyway, I would rather wear out than rust out."

Pain looked out of the corner of his eye, grinned and retorted with "Just saying Mr. Able Mind, that you may not be very balanced right now."

Able, feeling that Pain was going to give in to his request, pushed his advantage and hurriedly exclaimed "Never mind our mind! That's my job. I do the thinking; you do the work. Got it? Now let's get rolling!" So off they ran, to all the grand adventures that Able had waiting for them.

CHAPTER 2

12 Years later...

A frustrated Able, hurried down the path to catch up with Pain. "Hey, Pain, what's with the tendinitis in our ankles?"

Pain nonchalantly shrugged his shoulders and said, "It's just a warning. I'm starting to become weaker and can't keep giving you support like I used to."

Able tilted his head back and huffed out a deep and impatient sigh "Oh come on Pain! During our black belt training, we trained five or six days a week! Part of our every other day training, as you know, was comprised of one hour of hill running, 20 to 30 minutes of jump rope and calisthenics exercises, then 40 minutes of yoga and exaggerated stretching exercises. Then we spent another 45 minutes or so, every other day, lifting weights. We have been working out six to seven hours a week for 12 years, and now you're telling me that we're going to have problems with our body? Now? Are you serious?"

Pain chuckled sadly because he had braced himself for the impending tirade. He didn't say anything as Able poorly continued trying to convince Pain out of his decision.

Able flailed his arms in angry exuberance. "And that doesn't even count the karate tournaments that we prepared for and fought in! Remember we were not only competing in those tournaments but dominating the heavyweight division in the *35-years-old-and-up* age group. Although not really our age group overall; through a couple hundred sparring matches in the dojo against much younger opponents and over a dozen tournament matches, it's a fact that we were about 20 years older than our average competitor. But we did well, not only because of the hard work and cooperation but also because of our willing and able mind. That would be me, of course."

Pain rolled his eyes at Able's comment. As an afterthought Able added, "And thank you very much, for helping ceaselessly, Pain. You have been a real trooper through the tough and fun times. Like teaching at the karate school. That was so much fun! Even you would have to admit that"

Pain exasperatedly continued looking at the rocks as he continued down the path. "Nevertheless, Able, it wasn't easy at all. And it took about everything I had in me to help you." Pain paused and lightly grabbed Able's arm, turning him to look him determinedly in the eye. "Just to think, the only really painful situations we had occurred when we got our ribs smashed up in a tournament. And had to suffer from that for the better part of two years through all the training and tournaments. Although we were able to work through it, despite my reluctance." Able scornfully scoffed and started down the path again.

Pain followed and continued, feeling like he was trying to

deal with a mad man. "The only other major issue that we had was when we had that very severe neck and shoulder sprain/strain that our Jujitsu coach inflicted on us, seemingly trying to turn our head completely around when we were wrestling. What did he call that move he put on us? Oh yeah, a Brazilian necktie." Pain's tone turned wry and a little sour "Ha ha ha. Very funny. And of course, we could not work out for three weeks with that injury, even with intense physical therapy."

An annoyed look crossed Pain's face as he folded his arms across his chest. "Come to think of it, that was one of the few times that we took off from working out. Just 3 weeks in 12 years! Is it so hard for you to thank me, Mr. Able! Or should I call you, Mr. Ungrateful?" Practically shouted Pain.

To cover his discomfort at his brother's anger, Able placed an overly confident smile on his face. "I don't believe our run is anywhere near done or over, Pain. I think we might have slowed down a bit but can have a sensible and fitting workout program at least until 85 years old! Remember Jack LaLanne?"

Pain slowly blinked and came to a full stop. He felt his stomach roil at the thought of what his brother's idea of a "sensible work out" was for an 85-year-old.

Able still oblivious to Pain's reactions, continued down the path, chatting to himself. "I believe it will help us live that long if not longer. Remember, when we took that treadmill test a few years ago at the hospital for our yearly physical? Their graphs indicated that we had a cardiovascular system of a 21-year-old, even though we were 47 at the time! Man, we are doing good!"

Able's smile beamed in pride, as he watched Pain catch up with him and continued. "And our karate instructor said that our body fat was only about 12%. So, let's face it, we are in superb condition, and can continue to exercise at a nice clip for a long time." Able continued in a cocky tone spewing what his brother considered to be dribble. "In other words, although you'll never give me any of the credit, and try to take it all for yourself, it is my optimism that will allow us to live a long healthy life. I would appreciate it now if you would quit whining so much and give me a break. Can you do that?" Finished the now smug Able.

"Maybe I'll try." Responded the now cross Pain.

By the way, why are we starting to have these long bouts of tendinitis in our ankles when we run?" Able asked sincerely.

"I don't know, brother, what could have possibly caused it?" Pain answered with a question, sarcasm dripping from his tone. "Today its tendinitis, but tomorrow what will it be?" Pain shrugged his shoulders and firmly pointed to his mouth. "Read my lips: *my job* is to help us prevent damage to our body parts so that we can limit our suffering and misery in life and perhaps live longer."

Pain lowered his hand and shook his head. "Until now, I've never tried to take all the credit but make no mistake about it, as we get older, the focus is on me much more than you! We must make sure we have a healthy balance between our physical activities and fitness and being able to relax and enjoy physical comfort as long as we can. I acknowledge that you Able, our optimistic mind, has been responsible for much of our success in life to this point. But the times, they are a changing! You better pay attention to me, because as we get older, I become more useful, more dominant, with a bigger role, and a bigger voice between us."

Pain nodded to himself knowingly, and a nearly wild look came into his eyes. "In other words, I'm rising up! The civil war between us is just starting for all intents and purposes!" Pain pointed a finger to the sky, and borderline fanatically shouted. "I, Pain, body pain, am finally being elevated to my rightful place as the

leader, the savior, the righteous one, the victor! It took me long enough to realize this. But believe me, we've only just begun!"

Pain's voice dropped down to almost a growl. "Ignore me at your peril. If you do, you'll see, when all is said and done, I will completely kill off that optimism you have." Pain suddenly seemed to understand how far off tangent he went on. He straightened up a bit and cleared his throat.

With a brusque and business-like tone, Pain finished his thoughts with, "But I think it is necessary to save our life and make us happier. I will be the new hero. Now we can do this the hard way or the easy way, Able. Just don't make me have to torture you the way you tortured me." Able looked furtively out of the side of his eyes at Pain and awkwardly chuckled, not sure whether Pain was serious or not.

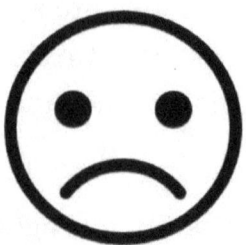

CHAPTER 3

The next day...

Able called out to Pain, "Let's go out and do some gardening!"

Pain growled back, "To hell with gardening today!"

Able put his hands on his hips and retorted, "You know Pain, I am concerned about your attitude lately."

Pain stopped, looked back and asked with a furrowed brow, "What are you talking about?"

Able folded his arms across his chest and started tapping his foot impatiently, then firmly stated, "We used-to-be able to come out and do the gardening without any problems from you. Now you have been tagging along and complaining more and more!"

Pain let out an angry huff and ground out, "Yes, because I am a sick and tired of you treating me like a nobody... like I don't matter."

Able barked out a harsh laugh. "Ha! Well, it's true. When I am mentally willing and able to do physical activity, I have always expected you to do what I have wanted to do. Mind over matter, you get it?" Able cruelly smiled at Pain and said. "So, in that way, you don't have any power or voice in my decision. It's always been that way, and always will. Again, you don't matter!"

Pain replied in a calm, matter-of-factually way, "Well, things are changing. I have decided to show you, to prove to you that I DO matter, and what you think in your mind doesn't matter anymore. I've had it with your endless optimism, day after day, year after year, while I suffer!"

Pain covered his eyes with his hand while shaking his head in disbelief. "I am tired and need rest more and more as we get older. It's not the mind over matter, it's that your mind does not matter from now on." Pain uncovered his eyes, pointed to his chest and adamantly said, "I, body pain, am the new sheriff in town... and if you try and ignore me, or belittle me, I will kill off your positive attitude and optimism."

For emphasis, Pain sent a quick bolt of pain through the body. "Enough is enough! I have had it with your arrogance! Always treating me as if I am useless and powerless. We do enough already. All you think about is you! Now I am going to show you that it is about us and that I am important too. If you don't respect me, you are going to pay for it, and the cost is hearing from me from now on. I am warning you!"

Able looked incredulously at Pain. "Warning me?"

Pain responded drolly, "Yes, stupid, I'm warning you! Although we have aged considerably, you don't demonstrate any wisdom. You think nothing changes with you and me over time, but you are dead wrong. Everything changes over time dummy. I am taking over!"

Able huffed a sigh and replied, "Well, since you want to fight, I might as well get this off my chest then. Did you notice when we went to the Doctor last week that the list of medical and health issues has grown? I hold you responsible for that. You are taking away our ability to have anywhere near a normal, or even semi-normal lifestyle." All the pent-up anger Able had been holding back, crept into his eyes. "What an a-hole you are. I am starting to really hate you! Inconsiderate bastard!"

Pain shouted in pure rage, "My fault?! You are such an idiot! You're to blame for our health problems and disabilities! You insisted on being strong and active. When I was at wit's end, telling you, pushing you and screaming at you to listen. And you were too selfish to understand that we needed to be a little less active before we became weak. And you didn't listen at all! Now we get to live with it! I dare you to believe that positive thinking crap when our body and life are completely falling apart." With tears of frustration welling up in his eyes, Pain cried out, "I hate you even more! You silly simple-minded clown! Something's got to change!"

Pain walked up to Able and stopped a few scant inches from his face and barked out a harsh laugh, jabbing his finger into Able's chest and continued, "And you are calling me inconsiderate. Ha! That's rich coming from you! Whatever happened to the golden rule? Do to others as you would have them do to you. You have totally forgotten to live by it! You disrespectful, hypocritical bum! You are hurting me Able..."

Pain backed up, shaking his head almost in defeat and said, "You are guilty of carelessly using up our bone density, joints, and muscle cells. You know we don't have an unlimited amount of those body parts. Also, we only have so much muscle fiber, and when it deteriorates, it never comes back."

Pain tried to reason with his brother one last time before it was too late. "I don't want to have limited mobility, or wind up completely disabled, do you? We might lose the independence we have always cherished. Imagine that! We might only be able to sit around and fuss and fight all day, just pointing fingers at one another as the one to be blamed for our dilemma. Like we are now! What kind of life would that be?" Pain wearily sat down on the edge of the path, and Able sat next to him, just as defeated and scared of the future. After a long while, the brothers got up and continued to wander down the path into their uncertain future.

CHAPTER 4

7 years later...

One day, after several more years had passed, the tired pair Pain and Able, plopped down on the edge of the path of life for a bit of a rest. Able pulled out their memory bank and sat stunned, looking over their memories. "I can't believe all of the health issues that we have had to deal with over the last seven years, starting with that seemingly minor case of tendinitis in the ankles! Who would've known then that it was just the beginning of our problems with pain and suffering: namely, the startling pain in the legs, knees, hips, lumbar, spine, and toes? And usually all day, with or without physical activity." Able shuddered, and Pain nodded.

Able continued where he left off, "Remember when bending over, walking up the stairs, minor gardening, or even walking made it so much worse? Often so debilitating over the years that all we could do is sit in a reclining chair or lie in bed to try and minimize it. I must be honest with you Pain, my normally optimistic mind became extremely pessimistic and overcome by SCREAMING, EXCRUCIATING PAIN." Pain woefully nodded his head.

"Also, the suffering caused by our other medical problems... the chronic fatigue, peripheral neuropathy, neuro-muscular damage, restless legs syndrome, high blood pressure, in-
somnia, the Parkinson's gait with stuttering and tremors. It was
almost too much, even without the chronic pain. Although I tried
to stay strong for us, I have lost more battles with you and Misery
than I can count. I'm so sorry I wasn't always there for you. I was
just beaten down, and... *It's been a living hell*!" Finished Able.

Pain put his arm around his shell of a brother's shoulders
and gently squeezed him to his side. Able looked up at Pain for
validation when he continued, "Since you were there, you know
Pain, that's not an exaggeration or hyperbole. It's hard for me to
believe that we made it this far! So often I thought we might not
make it, and honestly, sometimes I didn't want to live another
day with the terrible agony." Able tried to blink away tears that
threatened to spill over.

Pain shook his head in amazement. "I know Able. It's un-
believable. So many days were practically unbearable. And although I said and did a few things back in the day to try and scare
you so that I could finally be in charge, I had absolutely no idea
how bad things would get. I need you to believe that I wouldn't
wish what we've been through on my worst enemy. I just didn't
know how else to make you stop!"

Pain kept speaking to his brother consolingly, "I simply
wanted you to understand Able that we are, and always have been

in this together. Pain, real bad pain is equally as important, to want to do fun stuff! But for years I haven't stated my case well. I couldn't articulate when I was younger. Now I know how to make my presence felt. To make it clear that I am important too. We could have done this the easy way but no, we chose the hard way. You might be smart, but you are so slow in coming around and seeing things as they really are, instead of what you want them to be. I know how hard that is my friend because I am right here with you."

Pain placed a hand on Able's shoulder and looked him in the eye. "I also want you to understand Able that it is not nearly all my fault. It was also those negative statin side effects that caused most of our problems. And I'm very sorry for the role I played. Nobody deserves what you've been through mentally, or what I've been through physically for that matter. It is a true tragedy. I mean, come on, and I don't care how mentally tough you are, to have to endure so much physical and mental pain for so long. I think it's amazing that you've been able to keep your sanity! Fourth-degree black belt or not."

Able looked at his feet, trying to cover the tears welling up in his eyes. "Well, to be honest Pain, remember last year over those six weeks when we were bedridden? There is no doubt that we were having a nervous breakdown. I was so scared that I wouldn't be able to hold it together. It felt like we had post-trau-matic stress disorder (PTSD) because of the constant bombard-ment of medical problems for so long. It probably was the most difficult time we've ever had in life. That we get ambushed all... of... the... freaking... time! Just when we think it's safe to come out of the foxhole... BOOM! More pain, more fatigue, more medical problems."

Pain pulled Able into a hug and said. "I know. I was terrified and tried my best not to make it any harder on you. I really do love you Able, and for me not to care about you means that I don't care about myself."

Able pulled back and replied soggily, "Of course the worst part about it, over the years, is that we've tried everything to get better and alleviate having to suffer so much. Remember how our pain level averaged a seven for two and a half years, and for a couple of months, it was as high as 8 or 9. I know because I keep a daily log of our symptoms, called the Pain and Misery Index, where I calculated the daily and monthly index average, for almost three years. Wake up with pain and go to bed with pain. Never ending pain and misery, it seems. Always worrying about what the next day would bring."

Pain shook his head in disbelief again. "Yeah, and I didn't like to be in that wheelchair any more than you did. And to be officially classified as disabled! That's a label I still don't like at all. It's hard for me to see myself that way. Just think about it, all of the things we did to improve and live even a semi-normal life?"

Able scratched his head. "Well, to start with we have visited, discussed, or studied the findings of ten different doctors, with seven of them being specialists, just to understand and seek treatment for the newly discovered, but not well publicized, life-changing side effects of statins to some people. And found out that many athletes are intolerant to the drug."

Then Able started ticking off the things on his fingers. "What didn't we try between herbal remedies, acupuncture, massage therapy, body meditation, Tai chi, yoga, traditional meditation? When that didn't work, we tried Jacuzzi, sauna, light calisthenics, interval walking, plant-based diet, prescribed medication, self-medication, supplements, stress reduction. We were just trying to stay alive. It seemed we tried everything under the sun so that we could keep from hurting so, so bad."

Pain's face saddened again as he looked at his brother. "And the worst of it is, is that as tough as you are, there were many times that you wished we weren't alive. That YOU, of all people, considered suicide, not once, but many times because the pain and suffering was so overwhelming. And to be honest, it's understandable. But the truth is, I didn't want to die, or want you to die either. We were perfectly healthy and happy seven years ago, just loving life."

Able tried to lift the mood with his encouraging tone. "Well, at least we've had some relief from restless leg syndrome, so we can get some good sleep sometimes. And the Parkinson's disease symptoms have mostly gone away, so we don't usually have to walk with that gait anymore or have tremors and stuttering when we talk to people!"

Pain, feeling a little better, replied, "Yeah, I guess you're right. Remember, in our worst days we could never have any more than an hour and a half of physical activity each day. Which included walking up the stairs or doing simple tasks around the home, like light gardening or doing chores, without going through tremendous pain. Thankfully it has gotten somewhat better, but mostly because of that regiment of 12 supplements recommended in his book by that doctor who also has had awful statin side effects, very much like ours. And stress reduction. And proper treatment and medication, including pain management.

Able added, "Although it's terrible that the *apoptosis* has already killed a lot of our muscle cells. What did that one doctor tell us about the statin-induced *myopathy*?"

"That **your muscle cells are eating each other,**" Pain remembered and answered.

Able looked thoughtfully at Pain again, "And of course we still have to deal with the weak muscle cells, caused by *oxidative stress*. That we can't even go shopping sometimes without having to come home, get in the bed, and stay in it for a day or two because of fatigue is dreadful. Unfortunately, the pain and weakness get even worse with more physical activity and has caused us to be bedridden so often, occasionally for weeks or even a month at a time. But the worst part is that the frequency and severity are **totally unpredictable**, right? It absolutely sucks that we must limit our physical activity. And I don't want to!" Able let out a frustrated growl.

Pain looked sadly at Able and responded, "Are our medical problems ever going to go away? No, not likely. Most in the medical community feel that if the symptoms have not gone away by now, they probably never will." Pain's tone started dripping with sarcasm. "Boy, that's something to look forward to, right? Thanks, Statin manufacturers." Pain shook his head in disbelief. "How in the world do those folks sleep at night? Just to think! They are expanding their market now to include teens; surely pre-teens will be next. And then dogs, cats, horses. Why leave all that money on the table?!"

Able angrily kicked a pebble in the path. "And it sucks that we've had to cancel three nice vacation trips because pain and fatigue wouldn't allow us to go. That means we can't plan any more big trips; our traveling days are over. Or, do many other fun and enjoyable things either." Able sighed in utter depression. "Let's face it, we've gone from being strong and active to, in many cases, weak and inactive."

Pain replied in a placating tone, "Well, it's not quite as bad as all that now, Able. Although I realize that it used to be. At least now we can take light yoga and advanced art classes. Or play pool sometimes. Even take brisk walks occasionally; I remember when we couldn't do that. Not to mention the tap dance class over nine months, although we did have to sit out because of knee problems from time to time."

Able smiled hopefully. "It was fun doing that Jitterbug dance performance, because of our tap dance class, on a professional theater stage in front of a relatively large audience, don't you think?"

Pain nodded his head "Yes Able, it was kind of fun at the time. But look what we had to do to prepare for it and what happened afterward! Cortisone shots in both knees, massage therapy every week, and about 40 hours of practice and rehearsals. Unfortunately, I had to get more involved than I would've liked to, attempting to get you to understand we have our limitations. You only learn lessons the hard way."

Pain looked over and smiled, almost admiringly at Able. "I mean, you really don't know how to quit anything, Able. You **don't ever give up** and have always been that way. Sometimes that is good, but for this, it has been to our disadvantage. Most of my other friends learned moderation when they were in their youth. Even my best friends, Misery and Suffering, tell me that you are a hard case. Geez, why did I have to get a nut job as a brother? For once and for all, I am just trying to teach you balance."

Able rolled his eyes again. "Oh, you're such a pain! I can't be as bad as all that." Then Able looked into space, tapping his chin thoughtfully for a moment. "Yeah. But you might have a point Pain. It wasn't pleasant being on bed rest for six days after the theater dance performance was over. Or having our knee frozen stiff, because of inflammation, for three weeks."

Pain smiled sadly and nodded in agreement. "I'm not happy saying this, but... I told you so. I never did like that tap dance idea, and all the practice needed for the dance performance. Now we get to live with it. I just hope we get well soon. But next time you will listen, right?"

Able stared at Pain grinning saucily. "Will I?"

Pain raised an eyebrow with a wry grin on his face. "Won't you?"

EPILOGUE

I AM... Pain and Able. And so are you, sooner or later. Or you know someone who is struggling to live with pain, injury, or sickness on a day-to-day basis. It's a human condition. It is also very personal. We cannot feel or necessarily understand specifically what others are going through with their ailment or illness, even if we have been through a similar ordeal ourselves. But many of us can relate in general because we have experienced enough of our type of pain and/or sickness to know that having an adverse medical condition, or severe injury does affect our quality of life.

There are many reasons or perhaps hundreds of causes of our various afflictions. Everyone is different in one way or the other. And all our stories are unique and belong only to us. But one thing is the same about our struggle, regardless of the individual circumstances: **We feel it**, and **we own it**! As I said before, it's very personal!

My name is Kordye Turner, and I'm 62 years old. Here is my story; how I became so well acquainted with pain and suffering:

About 7 years ago, I began having problems with pain and soreness. The Health Maintenance Organization (HMO) that I am a patient of had recently increased the dosage of statin medication, but I did not see the connection at the time. When the pain continued and increased, I eventually went off the statin medication, hoping that doing so would alleviate the pain.

Meanwhile, the HMO kept insisting that I continue the statins. To say that the past seven years has been a nightmare is a fact rather than exaggeration. The only time that I've cried so much (other than from grief after my mother's funeral) has been in the last seven years. Much of the agony was caused by doctors' misdiagnosis, misunderstanding, and hostility toward me or the idea that statins were the cause of my medical problems. Often, I felt like a lone wolf crying in the wilderness.

My pain levels have ranged high constantly and were at their worst for about three consecutive years, during years three through five; in fact, pain levels ranging from 6-8 (with 10 being the highest level, and 1 the lowest) were normal for me. I even had back-to-back months where my pain levels averaged 9 one month, and 8 the next. The reason that I can be so precise with the numbers is that I kept an actual log, that I called a Pain and Misery Index, where I recorded in detail my medical symptoms on a day to day basis, and tallied the scores daily, weekly and monthly.

Simple activities like walking up the stairs, or bending over to put on my shoes, caused me terrible long-lasting pain. This was a drastic change from my former self, a person who spent about six hours per week exercising over 15 consecutive years, is a fourth-degree karate black belt, and prided myself on my gardening and handyman skills around the house. During my worst periods, I could no longer exercise or do any activity, including simply pruning my roses or walking around a store, for more than an hour and a half per day or I would end up writhing in pain all night.

My muscle cells were so weak that I sweated profusely even when I ate. I lost so much muscle mass that I am just a fraction of my former self now. Rather than seeing the future as bright and full of possibility, I have spent much of my time worrying about the pain and misery that tomorrow will bring. In the garage, I now keep a wheelchair handy for those times when I simply cannot walk.

During the first few years, the lack of support from doctors at the HMO meant that I never received adequate pain medication and had to spend a good portion of each day simply sitting in a chair or lying in bed in pain. At night, a very severe case of Restless Leg Syndrome (RLS) caused my legs to flail around uncontrollably and involuntarily (to be honest, sometimes the RLS symptoms were so strong and torturous that I would have preferred the pain). My toes are numb because of *peripheral neuropathy*, with sharp, jabbing, throbbing or burning pain at night.

Through research, I recognized that statins had caused me these problems and discontinued the medication. I hoped that the discontinuance of the statins meant that I could recover. This did not occur, and my symptoms continued to get worse. My arm and leg muscles have decreased substantially, and I am often completely overcome by fatigue. I often trembled, stuttered, and walked with a Parkinson's gait. The person who used to go on long walks with family and friends could only stand nearby and watch much of the time. My life became no longer active because of statins.

To me, it is outrageous that such negligence could have occurred in the modern world. That doctors do not teach the devastating consequences of statins, the most prescribed drug in the world, but instead, simply tout their effectiveness is astonishing.

It is unconscionable that doctors have not remained abreast of current research on the subject, which is voluminous and clearly states the horrendous consequences of taking statins, especially for those who exercise (for example, I just entered "statin side effects" in Google search and 21,100,000 results were posted; for "statin exercise intolerance" there were 5,220,000 results).

If a doctor's oath is to do-no-harm, then why have I and so many others been so horrifically harmed by statins??? It is my belief, based on the current deterioration of my health, that I will no doubt continue to deteriorate until I die or become fully debilitated physically or mentally from this illness (I was declared disabled five years ago) and regardless, HMOs and doctors will still push to sell statins without hesitation.

How I came to write this book, my first one ever was serendipitous. As I mentioned previously, after my dance performance, I went through a bout of fatigue leading to six days of bed rest and also had a frozen stiff knee for about three weeks because of severe inflammation. My karate instructor, Stuart Rowe of Pinole Karate, who is as much of a physical culturist than anyone that I have ever known, pleaded with me to stop all strenuous physical activity and exercise for a few months to give my body a chance to heal. He reasoned that I had tried just about everything else to rid myself of the pain and misery, and nothing else worked very much, with a couple of exceptions.

So, I promised my Instructor that I would take off at least one month. (It's hard for me not to do some type of exercise or workout because I would rather wear out than rust out!) Then I had to ask myself if I am not going to go to my fitness and yoga classes then what? Well, I had always been amused at the conversations that I had with myself over the last several years when it came time to decide whether I should do a particular physical activity, always weighing the pros and cons, and sometimes driving myself nuts. I had also concluded a while back that I knew enough about pain, sickness, and statin side effects to write a book about those subjects. So here it is!

I did not write the book for sympathy. And the book was not meant to be about me at its core. Instead, I wrote it for three good reasons: (1) help others that suffer from pain and sickness to understand and find comfort in knowing that we are all in the same boat, especially as we age, (2) provide a laugh for those of us who can relate to the Pain and Able internal struggle and conversations they have with each other as they go down the Journey of Life Road together. And (3) expose the damaging side effects of statins in the hope of helping others avoid my fate;
TO SAVE THE QUALITY OF LIFE AND POSSIBLY LIFE ITSELF FOR SOME INDIVIDUALS!!!

Statin side effects are generally kept hidden under the rug. But one study pointed out that about 10% of all people who take statins experience some type of side effects, even if it is only minor muscle pain or weakness. That proportion rises to at least 25% of people who regularly exercise and maybe 75% or higher among competitive athletes. (Source: Do Statins Make It Tough to Exercise, Gretchen Reynolds, NYT 3/14/2014.) That is why I needed to explain my background as an elite athlete in the story;

it wasn't to toot my own horn.

I mentioned before that there were a couple of exceptions that helped give me some relief: namely, taking Dr. Graveline's advice in his book <u>Statin Damage Crisis</u> after reading the book in the fifth year of my suffering. The book is excellent, and his analysis, in a nutshell, stated on the back cover is very accurate and revealing: "Now I have found the ultimate effect of statins on CoQ10 and dolichols is to damage the DNA of the mitochondrial life-force within our cells – mitochondrial mutation masquerading as **premature old age**."

He recommended taking a regiment of 12 supplements which would help me improve by striking at the root of the problem: damaged mitochondrial cells and neuromuscular nerve damage. The supplements, which I have taken religiously, did help noticeably. (By the way, I studied a lot of books and materials in an attempt to figure out and treat the cause of my medical condition, and think this is the one book that every doctor should read to understand and help patients with statin-induced myopathy and other related illnesses.)

The other reason for marked improvement to my health was from my primary care physician who told me to alleviate stress and rid myself of resentments, which I begin to focus on immediately. Believe it or not, before this advice, I had no idea that stress played such a major negative role in sickness, disease, and injury. Also, I found out later that mitochondria, the part of our cells that statins have the most impact on, is not only responsible for creating energy but also plays a key role in our *"multisystem biological response to stress.*"

Stress caused by illness and pain, also affects the mitochondria, which then has a negative impact on the rest of our biological functioning, such as insufficient heart energy and impaired cardio-vascular activity. This situation helps to explain why my blood pressure went from 120/80 consistently when I was working out and healthy to around 150 most of the time, and as high as 180 a few times before being recently prescribed two blood pressure medications. If it's not one thing, it's another with statin damage; Truly a vicious cycle!

I'm not going into detail here about the adverse side effects of statins, and there are many such as those explained in <u>Statin Damage Crisis</u> quoted below*. However, I have established a resource center for *Pain and Able Community* members and those who want to learn more. The website address is: www.pain-able.com

* "Tens of thousands of people have been victims of a vast array of statin drug side effects, ranging from permanent cognitive dysfunction and severe personality change to disabilities from peripheral neuropathy, permanent myopathy, and chronic muscular regeneration. It has been reported that muscle pain cases frequently become permanent and many neurologists now regard statin neuropathy as predictably resistant to traditional treatment. In addition to the crisis of thousands of people disabled by statin-associated neuro-muscular problems is the fact that **many physicians remain unaware that statins can even do this**."

◆ ◆ ◆

Lessons that I have learned during my experience and would like to share with you are:

- - *Study and know the side effects of all your medications personally*, don't assume anything. I made the mistake of believing the doctors when they told me or inferred that Statins were "perfectly harmless." Right. They damn near cost me my life and *did* cost me very important parts of my personal life.

- - *Find and keep a good doctor*. A quality physician can become your friend and savior. I really do feel that way about mine. The finest ones try their best to practice medicine with their coveted Hippocratic Oath in mind, and really do care! I've learned that if I treat them with respect and dignity, they'll do the same for me. Mutual trust is essential.

- - *Let your doctor know all your symptoms and exactly what you are suffering from*, to the best of your ability. Doctors are only human and make mistakes too by guessing! Help educate them.

- - Ensure that the medical community, including your doctor, works to *treat the root cause* of the medical problem, not just the symptoms. (Statin damaged victims must deal with this issue constantly because many in the medical community obviously can't treat a root cause that they fail to see, understand or accept).

- - Be persistent about your recovery. Keep an

open mind and *try different programs and treatments to help you improve.* Never stop fighting for your health; never settle.

- - *Saving lives or improving the quality of lives is the main point of medicine and doctoring.* When doctors help in this way, they feel good too! Believe in their better nature. Help them make a difference and not just a dollar.

- - Inform those around you if you have discovered the cause of your medical problems and possible cures and treatment tips. Share all forms of treatment and care that you have learned can help, even holistic and experimental ones. (If you had a remedy that provided cancer relief, for example, would you keep it to yourself?) I have found that *sometimes the best way to feel better is to help someone else feel better.*

  - Stay involved in internet and other communities that suffer from the same or similar afflictions. Be active learning from, teaching and supporting others who can relate to you and vice versa. *Have the courage to change the world, a little at a time, one person at a time.*

- - *Build a good team of people around you* that understand and can help treat your condition and provide support.

Thank you for taking the time to read this. I sincerely hope it helps you.

ABOUT THE AUTHOR

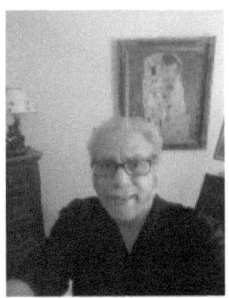

Kordye Turner is a retired businessman and investor. He holds a master's degree in business administration (MBA) from the Haas School of Business at UC-Berkeley, is a 4th-degree black belt in karate, enjoys oil painting, and has been a Civil War history buff since he was a boy.